I0456363

Dedication

This book is dedicated to the loving memory

of my mother and father,

Deborah and Larry

*Thank you for the joy and inner peace your
love continues to provide me every day,*

PEACE LIKE NEVER BEFORE

THE KEYS TO LIVING LIFE WITH PEACE OF MIND

D. L. Jones

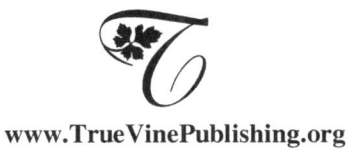

www.TrueVinePublishing.org

Peace Like Never Before
D.L. Jones

Published by True Vine Publishing Co
801 Dominican Dr.
Nashville, TN. 37228
www.TrueVinePublishing.org

Copyright © Deaderick Jones. All rights reserved. No part of this book may be reproduced, stored in a retrieval system or transmitted in any form or by any means, without prior or written consent of the publisher, except in the case of brief quotations, embodied in reviews and articles. Any person who does any unauthorized act in relation to this publication may be liable to criminal prosecution and civil claims for damages.

ISBN: 978-1-962783-49-1 paperback

ISBN: 978-1-962783-50-7 ebook

www.strategicsystems.org

Printed in the United States of America–First Printing

ACKNOWLEDGMENTS

My life, career, and this book are only possible because of special people, places, and experiences throughout my childhood, life, and career. These people, places, and experiences made it possible for these "key" principles of life to be shared with the world. I hope that none of you listed ever questioned your value or importance in my life. Thank you for making Lesson 18 possible!

From the beginning until now, a special thanks to…

- The Sitka Community of Milan, TN
- Carl Reed and Joslyn Allen Stewart
- The Baynham Family
- Mr. Hassel and the Metro Parks and Recreation Family
- Coach Peter J. Meadows
- The Brothers of Sigma Psi Omega, Inc.
- Mr. Bowers and the Whites Creek High School c/o 1994
- The A.I.T.F. Family
- The United States Navy, USS Patriot, and USS Scout

- Pastor Mike Whitsey
- The Prison Ministries
- The "at-risk" teens and families of the Juvenile Justice System
- The Bordeaux Church of Christ Family
- Mr. Howard Jones
- Mr. Ralph Thompson and Mr. Michael Tribue
- The students of Metro Public Schools, Nashville, TN
- Ms. Pamela Lee
- Bishop Joseph Warren Walker III and the Mt. Zion Family
- Keith and Nicole Mason, Venue 109
- The Homeless community and Room in the Inn
- Rev. Benjamin Sweat and the Mt. Bethel Family
- Refreshing Springs Church Family
- The Brothers of Kappa Alpha Psi Fraternity, Inc.
- Dr. Phara Fondren, Dr. Cynthia Croom, Lisa McCrady, and the Metropolitan Action Commission Family
- Jerome Thompson
- Terry David
- The Nashville Local Golfers Association
- The Men of "Father II Father", Nashville, TN

- The Men of "Men of Action", Salisbury-Rowan, NC
- The Men of "Fathers Strengthening Fathers", Greensboro, NC
- The North Carolina Head Start Association Family
- To my family and friends, you know how special our bond will always be!

And a very special thank you to my wife and sons for the inner peace your lives bring to me every day!

TABLE OF CONTENTS

Part V: Start With the Basics

Part VI: Feed Your Greatness

Part VII: When It's All Said and Done

INTRODUCTION

I have been blessed to work with countless individuals across the globe, representing diverse cultures and walks of life, and within these amazing experiences, I have uncovered a fundamental truth about the human experience: the secret to truly savoring life lies in achieving "peace of mind." This peace has the profound ability to transform your entire reality. When your mind is at peace, you become impervious to the turmoil around you. External events, opinions, and the fleeting judgments of others lose their power to unsettle you. With peace of mind, you navigate life's inevitable shifts with resilience, anchored by a mindset fortified with patience, tolerance, and clarity. This inner tranquility is the bedrock of a strength rooted not in external validation but in an absolute essence that the world cannot seize from you. It liberates you from the clutches of stress, anxiety, and worry.

There are times when it feels as if the world is spinning out of control, leaving you powerless. The chaos of our present reality might tempt you to believe that peace—or even the possibility of a sane existence—has become a distant memory. Yet, amid this disarray, contentment is not only possible but deeply attainable. There is an enduring belief in something greater, a transcendent force that offers "Peace Like Never Before."

In this book, I reveal hidden truths and time-honored principles that will allow you to experience a life marked by unprecedented peace. True "peace of mind" arises from a deeper comprehension and a re-framing of how life unfolds. It requires adopting a lens that sees beyond the immediate, that understands the subtleties of existence with a perspective shaped by wisdom. Throughout these pages, I will guide you in adopting key principles—accessible, yet pro-found—that transcend cultural and social boundaries, applicable to all regardless of background, race, or creed.

These timeless principles not only cultivate peace of mind but also tether you to your higher purpose, illuminating the path toward joy as you move through life. Allow these transformative concepts to influence your daily interactions and decisions, leading you to new discoveries that shape your experience of "Peace Like Never Before."

And always remember, nothing in our lives oc-curs by mere chance (a principle we will delve into in Part III). Your connection to this book, at this precise moment, is purposeful. So, prepare yourself for an extraordinary journey—a journey that will recalibrate your understanding of peace and lead you to a life of fulfillment and serenity that transcends circumstance.

Part I

LET PEOPLE BE PEOPLE

NOBODY'S PERFECT

It doesn't matter who you ask or where they come from—if they've spent any time in this world, nearly everyone seems to agree on one universal truth: "nobody is perfect." In a world rife with division and discord, it's a relief to know that we can still find common ground on such a fundamental principle. Yet, what's truly fascinating is that despite our collective recognition of human imperfection, we often fail to extend grace to others—and perhaps more tragically, to ourselves. There's a profound peace that arises when you master the art of allowing people to simply be human.

If we accept the truth that all human beings are flawed, it follows naturally that mistakes are inevitable. People, driven by varying circumstances and the ever-changing tides of life, often act or speak in ways that may not reflect their true essence or the person they might one day become. We are, after all, the cumulative result of trial and error, constantly evolving through learning and growth. Many of the mistakes we make could have been avoided, but each misstep is an opportunity to gain wisdom. If we can truly learn from each moment, including this very one, we find solace in the fact that we've survived—and that survival has armed us with insight for the future. But remember, wisdom is only as valuable as the extent to which you apply it.

Don't wallow in your mistakes. Allow yourself the grace to be human. It is in this acceptance that you begin to learn, grow, and transform. What you may view as a failure or misstep is often preparing you for larger moments and opportunities yet to come. There is no greater satisfaction than witnessing someone flourish after being given the space to be human. I am who I am today because key individuals in my life allowed me to make mistakes, to stumble, and to grow.

When you begin to navigate life with the understanding that everyone around you is at a different stage of their journey—each shaped by distinct influences, experiences, and choices—you're more likely to experience the peace that comes from letting people be themselves. You also develop the ability to meet people where they are without sacrificing your own sense of peace. This kind of understanding is profoundly healing, and it enables you to realize that no one's actions should dictate your inner calm. Instead, root your peace in principles that transcend human fallibility—principles that allow you to rise above the imperfections of others and yourself.

As you embrace this perspective, you'll unlock the ability to live a life grounded in peace—peace that is unshaken by the actions of others and fortified by the knowledge that mistakes are merely stepping stones on the path to growth. It is through this lens that you will come to understand what it means to live with "Peace Like Never Before."

Lesson #1
Reflections

_____

_____

_____

_____

_____

_____

_____

_____

_____

_____

_____

_____

_____

_____

_____

_____

_____

_____

TURN THE PAGE

It is difficult, if not impossible, to fully embrace the peace of today when your mind remains shackled to the past. Once something has transpired in our lives, it is an immutable fact—we cannot undo what has already been done. Our power lies not in altering the past but in deciding how much influence it will exert over our future. Friends, coworkers, spouses, and family members will inevitably disappoint or let you down, but remember: no one is perfect. We all stumble, make mistakes, and experience setbacks. The true key to inner peace is your ability to "turn the page."

Consider this example: Imagine you've just begun reading a 100-page book, and it starts off beautifully, captivating you. As you reach page 25, however, something happens that leaves you frustrated or upset. Do you abandon the book entirely because of this? Of course not. Instead, you "turn the page" and continue reading. As the narrative progresses, you find yourself enjoying it again, perhaps reaching page 50 where the story becomes engaging once more. Yet, inexplicably, you decide to flip back to page 25, reliving the frustration that page caused you. Despite being engrossed in the story on page 50, you allow the memory of page 25 to interrupt your enjoyment. You keep reading, but upon reaching page 75, you once again revisit page 25, replaying the same negative emotions.

Now, ask yourself: would anyone sensibly read a book in this manner? Of course not. And yet, many of us live our lives this way—allowing the "page 25" of our life, a painful event in the past, to steal away the peace and joy of the present. It is as though we assign more value to the experience of reading a book than to the experience of living our lives. Many people are unable to fully enjoy the peace of today because they continually allow a past event—their "page 25"—to influence their new day.

"Turning the page" is not about dismissing or overlooking what has happened. Rather, it is about choosing not to allow past events to dictate the peace and joy of today. Understanding that no one is perfect, that we all make mistakes, makes it far easier to "turn the page" and move forward. Life, much like a book, is written one day at a time. Each day is a sentence, each month a paragraph, and each year a chapter. In the end, your life's story may indeed have a difficult "page 25," but remember that the answer is not to give up—simply turn the page.

Forgive others, and just as importantly, forgive yourself. Reflect on the lessons that "page 25" has taught you, but do not let it dictate the pages yet to be written. The peace and joy of today deserve to be experienced without the weight of yesterday's burdens. So, turn the page, and allow yourself the freedom to embrace the new chapters of your life.

Lesson #2
Reflections

_____

_____

_____

_____

_____

_____

_____

_____

_____

_____

_____

_____

_____

_____

_____

_____

_____

_____

LEAVE THE LIGHT ON

Through years of working with people from all walks of life across the country, I have come to a profound realization: we all possess the capacity for love. However, it is in how we choose to express that love, and more specifically to whom we direct it, that our paths diverge. Throughout my career, I have worked closely with "at-risk" populations—individuals who have committed acts of robbery, kidnapping, assault, and even murder. Despite their transgressions, I have witnessed an unexpected truth: even those whom society might label as lost or irredeemable harbor deep wells of love for those they "choose" to care for. These same individuals, capable of horrific acts, can also be some of the most loving and nurturing people you'll ever meet if you are someone they decide is worthy of that love.

Yet, therein lies the complexity. Many of these individuals live their lives as if love is a switch to be flipped on and off, only activated when it suits them.

They expend energy throughout the day picking and choosing who is deserving of their affection, deciding in an instant when to show care and when to withhold it—much like dimming or extinguishing a light at will.

But here lies a transformative idea: what if, instead of rationing our love based on circumstance, we left the light on? What if we treated every encounter, regardless of the person's role in our life, with respect, kindness, and unconditional love? When we refuse to let external forces dictate our inner feelings—when we leave that light of love burning steadily—peace becomes our constant companion. It is impossible to live a peaceful life while viewing others as lesser, unworthy, or insignificant. Each person is imbued with inherent value, possessing unique gifts and potential. We must honor this in every interaction, knowing that doing so not only uplifts them but brings us closer to a deeper peace within ourselves.

Sustainable peace is rooted in consistency—the consistency of love, respect, and compassion. The more steadfast we are in letting that love flow freely, the less effort it requires to maintain our own inner tranquility. The act of turning love on and off throughout the day is emotionally exhausting; it requires us to navigate each situation with unnecessary caution and judgment. Instead, we should strive to keep the light on—to make love, care, and respect the default setting in every moment.

Try reminding yourself that no one is perfect. Decide today to leave the light of your best self shining brightly, not just for those you deem worthy, but for all. Life becomes remarkably easier, and infinitely more peaceful, when we abandon the exhausting practice of selective love. Leave the light on, consistently shining with love, valuing and respecting every person you encounter. In doing so, you will discover that life, when illuminated by love, becomes a peaceful journey rather than a chaotic struggle. Turn on the light of loving others, and let it shine—unceasing, unwavering, and full of peace.

Lesson #3
Reflections

_____

_____

_____

_____

_____

_____

_____

_____

_____

_____

_____

_____

_____

_____

_____

_____

_____

Part II

THE WORLD YOU CREATE

ART IMITATES LIFE

Although we all inhabit the same physical realm, the world as each of us perceives it is profoundly unique. Life, with its myriad variables, continually presents us with challenges and opportunities, and our peace and joy are inextricably tied to how we respond to these forces. The adage "art imitates life" resonates deeply here, and a handful of films over the years have masterfully illustrated the complexity of our existence. Life, at its core, is the product of how we process all that befalls us. And that processing is inherently linked to our perceptions of the world around us and the value we assign to the events we witness. The moment we grasp the fact that we are, in fact, co-creators of our reality, we open ourselves up to a peace previously unimaginable.

Take, for instance, *The Matrix*. In this cinematic masterpiece, a person is offered a choice: the "red" pill, which unveils a hidden reality governed by a new set of rules, or the "blue" pill, which maintains the illusion of the world as it is. By choosing the red pill, they unlock awareness of a deeper reality—a world within the world—where the individual, through belief in their intrinsic power, can "shift the atmosphere" around them. Similarly, many fail to experience peace and joy, not because of what is happening in their lives, but because of how they interpret those happenings. They neglect to wield their uniqueness, their ability to alter the energy around them. The world is constantly in flux, bombarding us with shifts and changes, but we must never forget that we retain the power to determine how much of that external chaos will truly affect us.

It is not necessary to respond to everything the world throws at us. To do so would be akin to chasing the wind, an endless and exhausting pursuit of things beyond our control. Without mastering the art of selective engagement, the world dictates our thoughts, actions, and ultimately, our inner peace. To have peace in the midst of life's storms does not imply ignoring reality; rather, it grants the mental space to process events with calm deliberation.

Consider a ship at sea. There is nothing inherently problematic about a ship being in the water, but trouble arises when the water gets inside the ship. So too in life: while we must exist in this world, we must vigilantly guard how much of the world we allow into our minds. Each day, we are presented with a choice—a choice to determine which variables will foster our inner peace, and a mandate to protect our minds from the incessant demands of the external world. By anchoring ourselves in key life principles (Lesson 13) and consistently affirming our ability to shift the atmosphere (Lesson 12), we cultivate the resilience to weather life's storms with grace.

Lesson #4
Reflections

_____

_____

_____

_____

_____

_____

_____

_____

_____

_____

_____

_____

_____

_____

_____

_____

_____

_____

HAPPINESS IS A CHOICE

There is something profoundly soothing about the sound of birds chirping at dawn, a gentle reminder that a new day has begun. It's remarkable how these creatures, oblivious to the uncertainties of the future, still manage to fill the air with their joyful songs. It almost seems as though the birds make a deliberate choice to be happy, to sing in spite of the unknown. In doing so, they not only revel in their existence but also spread joy to others, never allowing the unpredictability of tomorrow to silence their song. In much the same way, we too have the power to choose happiness intentionally.

One of the reasons people struggle to find lasting happiness is that they often tether it to fleeting or material things—things that are by their nature inconsistent. When happiness is bound to external circumstances, it becomes as unpredictable as the tides, rising and falling based on the whims of the world. To experience enduring happiness, however, one must master the art of choosing to be happy deliberately, irrespective of external conditions.

Consider this scenario: A woman orders a pair of shoes she's been eyeing for quite some time, patiently waiting for the price to drop. At last, she gets the deal she hoped for and places the order, only to be informed that the shoes will take 4-6 weeks to arrive. Despite the delay, the moment she hangs up the phone, she is immediately filled with joy, even though the shoes are still weeks away.

In this example, her happiness is not contingent on the actual arrival of the shoes, but rather on the expectation of them. She has chosen to be happy in the moment, not because of any certainty that the shoes will indeed arrive, but because of what she believes will happen in the future. If something as simple as shoes can elicit this kind of anticipatory joy, how much more deserving is your life and its limitless possibilities of that same intentional happiness?

We are all familiar with what happiness feels like, but to root it in something deeper—such as your gifts, talents, and life's purpose—frees you from the volatility of external events. By anchoring your joy in the more meaningful aspects of your existence, you gain clarity to recognize and resist the forces that seek to rob you of your happiness. This deliberate choice allows you to experience a peace and joy that the world cannot take away, a happiness that is resilient and unwavering in the face of life's uncertainties.

Lesson #5
Reflections

_____

_____

_____

_____

_____

_____

_____

_____

_____

_____

_____

_____

_____

_____

_____

_____

_____

_____

HINDSIGHT IS 20/20

The familiar adage "hindsight is 20/20" speaks to the clarity we often gain when reflecting on past experiences. When we look back on certain moments in our lives, we can discern where things fell into place and where we might have chosen a different path. But more importantly, hindsight often reveals the countless times we were overwhelmed by stress, anxiety, or worry—times when inner peace eluded us. If we're honest, many of those days we spent in turmoil were ones we could have enjoyed more fully, savoring the richness of life instead of succumbing to fear or doubt.

Hindsight is not just a window into our past but a teacher for our present. It should prompt us to make a deliberate choice: to never again allow ourselves to be robbed of happiness. As we explored in Lesson #5, happiness can be a conscious decision. Learning from our past means basing our joy on deeper, more meaningful aspects of life, rather than the fleeting or unpredictable circumstances that surround us.

Consider, once more, the birds. They have nothing stored up for the future—no guarantee of what the next moment will bring—yet they still sing, fully immersed in the present. They embrace the day and the joy it offers, refusing to allow life's uncertainties to steal the opportunity to be who they are meant to be. If the birds allowed themselves to be consumed by worry or stress, they would miss out on the beauty of the day and the connection they offer to the world around them. Likewise, when we let our circumstances paralyze us with fear, we too miss precious moments and opportunities that life is offering right now.

Take, for example, a scenario involving a cruise ship that encounters a fierce storm. As the ship is battered by the weather, parts begin to break apart. The Captain, after assessing the damage, assures the passengers that they will reach shore safely in a few days. As the storm intensifies the following night, some passengers cling to the Captain's words, eating and resting peacefully, while others contemplate jumping ship or go without sleep, gripped by fear. By the third day, the storm subsides, and the ship arrives safely at shore.

Although all the passengers ultimately make it to

shore, their experiences differ drastically. Some passed the time in peace, while others were consumed by worry and fatigue. This example illustrates the essence of mastering life's storms: while challenges and uncertainties will come, your experience of them is shaped by your mindset. The goal is to reach a point where, when life's storms rage around you, you can still anchor yourself in the knowledge that the storm will pass. You will endure, and in the meantime, you can continue to live, to enjoy the moments and opportunities that each day brings.

Reflect on your past and let it guide you towards a deeper calm. Let it teach you to meet today's challenges with an unshakable peace, knowing that you have survived before and will again. Life's uncertainties need not strip you of joy; instead, they can be the very reminder that, even amid the storm, there is still beauty to be found and moments to be lived.

Lesson #6
Reflections

_____

_____

_____

_____

_____

_____

_____

_____

_____

_____

_____

_____

_____

_____

_____

_____

_____

_____

_____

_____

ROUTINES AND CHECK-INS

E ach day we awaken, we are confronted with a flood of thoughts, tasks, and agendas, pulling us in multiple directions. Attaining a peace that surpasses understanding requires a deliberate and mindful effort. It begins with the conscious decision to take control of your day by intentionally setting routines and benchmarks that ground you in the awareness of your own "world"—the world you are creating within—and your active pursuit of peace. At the very start of the day, you must make a resolute choice to focus on peace and joy as your ultimate goals. From that point forward, it becomes an exercise in not allowing yourself to be consumed by the ever-changing currents and challenges that will inevitably arise throughout the day. The mental discipline required to remain aware of the constantly shifting world around you demands intentionality.

Just as no one embarks on a journey without checking mile markers or stopping at checkpoints along the way, navigating the complexities of a single day requires similar vigilance. With the world throwing countless distractions and challenges your way, it is essential to set up mental benchmarks throughout the day—moments where you remind yourself of the peace and joy that are yours for the taking. If you own a cell phone, try setting alarms or reminders at various points in the day, each one acting as a gentle nudge to refocus on the goals you've set for yourself. Simple reminders like, "Stay Focused," "Don't React," or "Peace on Purpose" can serve as powerful anchors amid the chaos. Schedule these alerts for morning, noon, and evening, ensuring that as the day unfolds, you are periodically reminded that your peace originates from within, not from the external world. You choose to live a life grounded in what truly matters, starting with the decision to not be overwhelmed by whatever life presents.

Reflect back on Lesson 4, and remember to be mindful of the world you create. There was a time when knowing the thoughts of everyone around you was a distant, almost unimaginable concept. Yet now, with the advent of social media, it has become commonplace to encounter the thoughts, opinions, and emotions of thousands of people in a single day. Constant exposure to this flood of external stimuli makes it increasingly difficult to maintain inner peace and keep joy at the forefront of your life. How can one cultivate true peace when bombarded by the endless stream of other people's viewpoints and their personal definitions of happiness? Meanwhile, as individuals pour time and energy into gaining "likes" and "views" from strangers, they risk missing the real connections and peace that could be nurtured in their immediate, real-world relationships.

The act of setting intentional checkpoints and daily reminders ensures that you create space to reset from the inevitable disruptions that life will bring. Without these deliberate moments of pause, you risk becoming a victim of life's demands, reacting to every external trigger. By establishing reminders throughout your day, you reaffirm your commitment to maintaining the peace and joy that is available to you in the present moment. These reminders also serve as a beacon, guiding you through the noise and reminding you of your conscious decision not to be swayed by the things happening in the world around you.

Lesson #7
Reflections

_____

_____

_____

_____

_____

_____

_____

_____

_____

_____

_____

_____

_____

_____

_____

_____

_____

_____

Part III

NOTHING JUST HAPPENS

SEIZE THE MOMENT

Life takes on an entirely new dimension when you come to the profound realization that nothing in it just happens by chance. When you grasp that every occurrence in your life, whether significant or seemingly trivial, carries meaning, you begin to see the value in each moment. Even your mistakes, those moments you wish you could undo, happen for a reason. If you've made it through and are still standing, those mistakes were not in vain. They are lessons, chapters in the book of your life, waiting for you to extract their wisdom and use it to write the next, more enlightened pages of your story. All that's left is for you to seize the moment right in front of you.

Seizing the present moment is deeply intertwined with mental well-being. Our minds often drift—either toward the future, where uncertainty breeds anxiety, or back to the past, where regret or nostalgia can spark depression. Yet, the true key to inner peace lies in freeing your mind from the shackles of both the future and the past. By doing so, you can fully inhabit the present, where mental clarity and well-being thrive. The act of being present allows you to live with a heightened awareness of today, embracing life as it unfolds right now.

You have only one mind, and when that mind is preoccupied—whether with the lingering shadows of the past or the imagined possibilities of the future—you inevitably miss the richness of the present. You cannot be mentally present while simultaneously dwelling in another time. Life is not meant to be lived constantly in the memories of what once was, no matter how sweet or painful those memories might be. Instead, seize the opportunity to create new memories, to write new chapters today. Life is like a book, with each day offering the chance to craft a new sentence, a new page. Don't let the page of today remain blank because you were too consumed by thoughts of yesterday or tomorrow.

I've experienced profound revelations because I embraced the idea that "nothing just happens." It allowed me to seize the moments as they unfolded, knowing each one held significance. Once you internalize this truth—that nothing in your day is random, and that being present is the most powerful way to live—you open yourself up to peace like never before. It's about being here, fully attentive to the lessons and opportunities life is offering you right now. Free your mind from the clutter of overthinking, and give yourself the gift of experiencing the newness and richness of today.

There is immense peace in knowing that you are mentally available—ready and willing to engage with the special moments and opportunities each day presents. Let go of the past and stop obsessing over the future. Instead, live fully in the now, and seize the life in front of you, because this is where the real magic happens.

Lesson #8
Reflections

_____

_____

_____

_____

_____

_____

_____

_____

_____

_____

_____

_____

_____

_____

_____

_____

_____

_____

_____

GROWING WITH SCARS

Have you ever paused to truly appreciate the beauty of a fully mature tree? There's one that has stayed with me throughout my life and career, a constant reminder of strength and resilience. Day after day, I would glance out the window, captivated by its grandeur, its steadfastness. One afternoon, I felt compelled to walk closer, to stand beneath its branches and savor the cool shade it provided. But as I approached, I noticed something new: the tree bore the marks of its journey. There were broken limbs, deep scars from cuts, and signs of the battles it had faced—years of storms and harsh weather etched into its bark. Yet, despite all these imperfections, the tree remained strikingly beautiful.

In much the same way, as we go through life, we inevitably collect scars—visible and invisible reminders of the challenges we've faced. These scars, though, are not the final word on our lives. They are part of our story, but they do not define our beauty or the success we are capable of achieving. Living in this world means we will encounter people and circumstances that may leave lasting marks, often unpredictable and out of our control. Yet, just as the tree stands tall and whole despite its wounds, so too can we continue to grow, thrive, and remain beautiful in the face of adversity.

What's more, these scars—the very things we sometimes wish we could erase—are often integral to our beauty and strength, particularly when we align ourselves with our true purpose. In fact, those very scars can become the reason for our success, the driving force behind our purpose, gifts, and talents. No matter what trials you've faced, nothing has the power to diminish your capacity for greatness or fulfillment. That oak tree I admired was still magnificent, still providing shade and shelter. Its scars, while visible up close, didn't detract from its essence; if anything, they deepened my appreciation for the tree's resilience. And so it is with our lives—our scars do not detract from who we are or who we can become. For those who take the time to see us up close, those marks of endurance only enhance our value and significance.

In fact, it is precisely because of the scars in my own life that I've been able to help others find their own peace and strength. These marks are not just symbols of hardship, but of survival, wisdom, and beauty. May you come to find a peace that surpasses understanding, recognizing that your scars are not barriers but badges of resilience. Like the great tree, your beauty remains, undiminished by the challenges you've faced, ready to be appreciated by those who truly see you.

Lesson #9
Reflections

_____

_____

_____

_____

_____

_____

_____

_____

_____

_____

_____

_____

_____

_____

_____

_____

_____

_____

_____

As a Man Thinketh

How you perceive yourself has an indelible impact on the trajectory of your life. Your belief in your own abilities is the foundation upon which every pursuit is built. If you don't believe you can accomplish something, you won't even take the first step toward it. As Henry Ford said, "He who says he can, and he who says he can't are both usually right." Everything that unfolds in your life, whether positive or negative, is a direct result of what you've told yourself. Before any action is taken, it is first conceived in the mind. This holds true across all aspects of life: as a person thinks, so shall their life become. The key, then, is to truly see and know your own worth, for only then can you experience the peace that naturally flows from such self-awareness.

Imagine, for a moment, ten one-dollar bills. Now, picture these bills like the characters in those M&M commercials—animated, with the ability to talk and express themselves. These ten dollar bills head to a store, where they find an item priced at exactly one dollar. However, one of the dollar bills chooses not to get in line, feeling unworthy to make the purchase, all because of what it has endured on its journey to the store—perhaps it's wrinkled, torn, or a little worn from life's experiences. It's disheartening to witness that one-dollar bill not recognize its inherent value, despite being just as capable of making the purchase as the others.

This is often how people operate in life. We all have the same intrinsic value and the same potential for greatness. Yet, some of us fail to see it because of the hardships we've endured. It is equally as saddening when someone reaches a point in life where they no longer recognize their worth or their ability to achieve what others can. The truth is, our value never diminishes, regardless of what we've been through. We are born with a unique "fingerprint"—a distinct identity and purpose that cannot be replicated (we'll dive deeper into this in the next lesson). The key is to believe in yourself enough to put yourself in the position to unlock your full potential. Once you truly acknowledge your value, you position yourself to experience a peace that comes from within.

There is a profound peace in knowing that you are equipped to share your gifts with the world. When you allow yourself to see that every experience—both the triumphs and the challenges—has prepared you for what lies ahead, you open the door to a deeper sense of peace. This peace becomes an integral part of your journey toward realizing your potential and fulfilling your purpose. But this peace cannot manifest unless you first believe it is possible. Each day presents countless choices, and you can choose to walk in a peace that transcends the understanding of those around you. However, it all starts with you telling yourself that such peace is within reach. Without that belief, it will never become a reality.

Lesson #10
Reflections

_____

_____

_____

_____

_____

_____

_____

_____

_____

_____

_____

_____

_____

_____

_____

_____

_____

_____

_____

Part IV

UNDERSTANDING YOUR UNIQENESS

USE YOUR FINGER PRINT

It's always a breath of fresh air when we encounter a universal truth that resonates with all of us—something so undeniable that it unites us in its simplicity. One such truth is the uniqueness of our fingerprints. Each one of us carries a fingerprint that is unlike any other, past or present. But here's something even more powerful: your uniqueness goes far beyond the ridges on your fingertips. Just as your physical fingerprint is one-of-a-kind, so too is your set of gifts, talents, and the purpose you were meant to fulfill on this earth.

You have a distinctive role in the world—gifts and talents that are yours alone to bring to life. No one else can accomplish what you are meant to do, and it's this irreplaceable essence that makes your life as valuable as anyone else's. These inherent abilities are not only part of what makes you special, but they are also integral to your daily sense of peace and fulfillment. When you nurture your gifts and talents, much like watering a plant, you cultivate a life filled

63

with joy and purpose (we'll explore more on how to feed this greatness in Lessons 16 and 17). But it all begins with the belief—an unshakeable knowing—that just as you have a fingerprint, you have something extraordinary within you.

This understanding is crucial because, while there are universal principles that guide us toward success, the path to your success will always be uniquely yours, tailored to your distinct talents and gifts. You don't have to follow the blueprint laid out by others to achieve greatness. If that were the case, the world would never evolve. You are meant to embrace your individuality, to lean into your uniqueness, and leave a lasting impact through the gifts and talents that only you possess.

So, trust in your fingerprint, not just the one on your hand, but the one written into your very being. Use your talents, your gifts, and your purpose to shift the atmosphere around you. Don't allow the world to define you. Instead, embrace the peace and joy that come from knowing you have something remarkable to offer—a contribution to the world that no one else can make.

Lesson #11
Reflections

_____

_____

_____

_____

_____

_____

_____

_____

_____

_____

_____

_____

_____

_____

_____

_____

_____

_____

_____

_____

No Limitations

Many people miss out on the peace and joy of today because they let the world around them dictate who they are and what they can become. But remember, you are unique. You have a set of gifts and talents that are entirely your own, just like your fingerprint. It's important not to let life's circumstances or the world around you impose limitations on your potential. Life becomes much more fulfilling when you embrace who you are, free from restrictions. Living without limitations allows you to experience peace and joy—not because of what's happening around you, but because you've chosen to be the best version of yourself, regardless of the atmosphere or challenges you face.

When you limit yourself based on your surroundings, job description, or external expectations, you allow those factors to control your outcomes and hinder your growth. Imagine, instead, using your gifts whenever the opportunity arises—not just when you're paid for it. When you do this, you begin to see your gifts make room for you in life. The peace that comes from being your authentic self while positively impacting others will bring deep satisfaction. Eventually, the right person at the right time will recognize your talents. Until then, take joy in the peace that comes from fully using your gifts each day.

Much of your success in life will be tied to others recognizing the value you bring now. That's why it's crucial to seize every chance to use your talents. Don't let the world or your environment dictate when or how you express your gifts. Instead, choose to live without limitations and experience the freedom that comes with being 100% yourself. When you do this, you won't remain stagnant. Remember, you possess something that no one else on earth can offer. The world will only see that uniqueness if you live without limiting your gifts and talents.

Living without limits provides the time and space for your gifts to grow and flourish, allowing you to reach your full potential. It also enables you to make the most of your current circumstances. Your gifts and talents can influence the atmosphere around you, and by embracing them, you can change the world instead of letting the world change you.

Consider the example of Chris, a man with a

natural talent for building, who was falsely accused and sent to prison. Despite his situation, Chris didn't let his environment or circumstances limit him. When a construction project in the prison seemed unsolvable, he used his talents to complete it effortlessly. Little did he know, one of the prisoners observing his work was a wealthy construction business owner about to be released. This man, impressed by Chris's skill, offered him a job once Chris was released. Chris, later found innocent, contacted the businessman and was immediately placed in charge of major projects.

Why did this happen? Because Chris refused to let his surroundings dictate who he could be. He didn't allow his circumstances to hold him back, and by continuing to use his gifts, he unlocked new opportunities for success. The same holds true for you. A significant part of your peace and joy comes from being your authentic self without limitations. Let your gifts and talents guide your path, and you will find the peace that comes from living fully through them.

Lesson #12
Reflections

_____

_____

_____

_____

_____

_____

_____

_____

_____

_____

_____

_____

_____

_____

_____

_____

_____

_____

Part V
START WITH THE BASICS

AFTER THAT, THERE'S NOTHING ELSE

Life presents many challenges, and the longer we live, the more they seem to pile up. However, one essential truth remains: without having the core elements of your life in alignment, finding peace and joy in other areas will always be difficult. A peaceful and joyful life starts with understanding that no matter who you are, your life has a purpose beyond what the world or others may present to you. Your purpose isn't just about personal success—it's tied to the well-being and success of others beyond yourself. Recognizing and walking in this purpose is a key to unlocking true peace and joy.

It's easy to get distracted by the many options and opportunities life offers, but those distractions can lead you away from your true purpose. I'm reminded of a letter my father wrote to me before he passed away. It was filled with wisdom, so much so that I didn't know where to begin. But in the last line of the letter, he made it simple: "Take a look at your family photo. After that, there's nothing else :-)." With this, he was telling me that, despite all the complexities of life, if I remembered my basic purpose—represented by my family—everything else would fall into place.

In today's world, it's easy to lose sight of that basic purpose. The world often tries to make us define our value by external achievements and distractions. But peace and joy come from focusing on those who truly value us and celebrate our presence, words, and thoughts. Start with the basics: focus on the people who matter most to you and allow them to be the foundation of your peace and joy. The happiness and fulfillment you gain from being present and supportive for those who love you will naturally spill over into other areas of your life.

When you start with your basic purpose in life, everything else becomes clearer. Those fundamental relationships—whether with family, close friends, or those who depend on you—become the source of your peace and joy. By prioritizing these relationships, you'll find that other areas of life that once caused stress or stole your peace will start to fade away. You'll be so focused on your natural purpose that there won't be space left in your mind for the distractions and worries that used to weigh you down.

Peace and joy become easier to maintain when you're fulfilling your natural purpose, especially with those who appreciate and value you the most. It's in the basic acts of showing up for those who count on you that you'll find a deeper sense of fulfillment. When you take care of those most important to you, your mind becomes freer, and the daily challenges that once seemed overwhelming lose their power to disturb your peace.

In the end, peace and joy are the natural fruits of living a life centered around your purpose. When you're in tune with your natural role in life—caring for those you love and fulfilling your responsibilities—the peace you seek will follow. You won't be distracted by unnecessary thoughts or burdens because your mind and heart will be focused on what truly matters. Start with the basics of life, and everything else will follow. The peace and joy that come from fulfilling your purpose will be unlike anything you've experienced before.

Lesson #13
Reflections

_____

_____

_____

_____

_____

_____

_____

_____

_____

_____

_____

_____

_____

_____

_____

_____

_____

_____

_____

YOU GOT A TRAIN

A father bought his young son a train set, which delighted the boy so much that his parents had to keep the train running until it naturally slowed down. A few days later, while his mother was cooking breakfast, the boy became irritated and upset. His mother asked him why he was crying, despite having the train. The boy, upon being reminded of his cherished train, looked at it with renewed joy and appreciation, forgetting his frustration.

In life, it's easy to get caught up in challenges and changes, leading us to forget the things we once cherished and were grateful for. If you're reading this book, you likely have much to be thankful for, including things you may have forgotten to appreciate. When you focus on gratitude and enjoy the good aspects of your life, there's less room for stress and anxiety over things beyond your control.

Personal Example: I remember the first holiday season without my parents. I went to their graves to mourn, and as I walked, I heard the cheerful sounds of Pre-K music. I saw two parents pretending to interact with their child who had passed away. At that moment, I thought of my sons at home and realized, "You've got a train!"

That realization shifted me from mourning to gratitude. I was thankful for my living sons and for the time I had with my parents, which provided me with valuable life lessons I can now share with others. No matter what you're facing, you have your own "train" if you take a moment to recognize it. Even something as simple as being able to read this book is a sign of having blessings to be grateful for. Many people would love to have the things you do. Embrace gratitude and focus on the positive aspects of your life, and you'll find peace and joy.

Lesson #14
Reflections

_____

_____

_____

_____

_____

_____

_____

_____

_____

_____

_____

_____

_____

_____

_____

_____

_____

_____

ONE DAY AT A TIME

U nderstanding the importance of taking life one day at a time can lead to unprecedented peace. Each new day brings a chance to apply lessons from the past while presenting its own set of challenges. Just as previous days have passed, so will this day, regardless of what it holds.

There will be moments when focusing solely on making it through the day is all you need, and that's perfectly okay. Life often becomes overwhelming when we try to solve everything at once or worry about the future instead of handling today's challenges. There's no need to have all the answers for tomorrow right now. By focusing on today, you can appreciate the present moment and avoid missing out on its beauty.

Many people have struggled or given up on life due to the overwhelming nature of their circumstances. However, reminding yourself to take life one day at a time can alleviate some of that stress. Each day offers new strengths and opportunities, and by concentrating on what's important today, you can better manage other variables life presents.

Taking it one day at a time is easier when you intentionally avoid anxiety about the future and depression about the past. By being present, you open yourself up to the opportunities of today and can engage more meaningfully with those around you. This approach allows you to reflect on the day's lessons and appreciate the moments you have.

Living each day as if it's your last encourages you to make the most of your time with others. Reflect on those who are no longer here and consider if they spent their last day worrying about the future. Don't let that be your story. Start making a deliberate effort to embrace each day fully, seizing every moment and cherishing those around you. There is a deep inner peace available to you in the present moment.

Lesson #15
Reflections

_____

_____

_____

_____

_____

_____

_____

_____

_____

_____

_____

_____

_____

_____

_____

_____

_____

_____

_____

_____

Part VI

FEED YOUR GREATNESS

LIONS, GAZELLES, AND BABOON MEAT

Experiencing peace like never before is possible when you see your life's steps as part of a greater journey and connect your current actions to your dreams and aspirations. When people lack focus or direction, they often settle for whatever is convenient, losing sight of their true potential. To achieve inner peace, it's essential to bring your dreams from the realm of imagination into clear sight.

Example: In the jungle, a lion wakes up each day with a gazelle on his mind. Although he sees the gazelle in the distance, the path to it is obstructed by the jungle. Despite the distance, the lion's focus sharpens, and he feels a renewed sense of purpose. Knowing the gazelle is within sight, he refuses to settle for less, such as eating baboon meat along the way. Every step he takes towards the gazelle counts, and the sight of his goal provides him with inspiration and strength.

The lion's life changes dramatically once the ga-zelle is in sight. His focus is clear, and each step he takes is purposeful, leading him closer to his goal. This focus prevents him from settling for less. Simi-larly, when you have a clear vision of your dreams, you remain motivated and less likely to accept medi-ocrity.

Without a visible goal, many people settle for less, just as the lion might have eaten baboon meat if the gazelle had not been in sight. By setting your sights on your dreams and understanding the impor-tance of each step, you will find greater peace and purpose. Allow yourself to envision your goals and take deliberate steps towards achieving them, know-ing that each step counts in the pursuit of your dreams.

Lesson #16
Reflections

_____

_____

_____

_____

_____

_____

_____

_____

_____

_____

_____

_____

_____

_____

_____

_____

_____

_____

_____

_____

_____

VISION TO SEE

You can achieve a profound sense of peace of mind about your dreams, whether you're actively pursuing them or not. Just as a lion finds focus and peace when he spots a gazelle, you can harness the power of your dreams, gifts, and talents to guide you. Bringing these dreams from your mind into reality is entirely feasible in today's world.

In the past, people created vision boards to visually represent their goals and aspirations. These boards served as daily reminders of their desired outcomes, helping them stay focused despite the obstacles they faced. Your dreams and aspirations are a reflection of where your gifts and talents can take you, and using a vision board can keep you attuned to your goals without being bogged down by life's barriers.

Today, creating a vision board is easier than ever. You no longer need physical materials like glue and magazines. Instead, you can simply search the internet for images that represent what you want to achieve and save them on your phone or computer. Even if you can't display them on a physical board, having these images easily accessible allows them to serve as your personal gazelle. They keep you focused on your goals and prevent you from settling for less.

These saved images or vision boards help guide your decisions, ensuring that each step you take brings you closer to your dreams. By keeping your aspirations in sight, you maintain motivation and avoid falling for less satisfying options. Each day, as you take steps toward your goals, you can experience a deeper peace knowing you are progressing.

Regardless of where you are in life, let your dreams and aspirations become your primary focus. Avoid settling for less and allow your vision board or saved images to inspire and guide you. By staying determined and taking one step at a time towards your goals, you will find inner peace and strength similar to a lion with a gazelle in sight. Embrace your unique gifts, believe in your potential, and let your vision board be a beacon guiding you to your dreams.

Lesson #17
Reflections

_____

_____

_____

_____

_____

_____

_____

_____

_____

_____

_____

_____

_____

_____

_____

_____

_____

_____

_____

WATER YOUR GREATNESS

The Chinese bamboo tree is renowned for its astonishing growth, reaching up to ninety feet tall in just six weeks. However, this rapid growth is preceded by a hidden, five-year period during which the tree appears to do nothing but grow underground. During this time, consistent daily watering is crucial; missing even a single day can jeopardize the progress made over the years. The farmer must remain diligent, continually watering with the vision of the towering tree in mind.

Similarly, your greatness and potential require daily nurturing. Just as the bamboo tree needs persistent watering, your gifts and talents need consistent care and attention. Although it was once more challenging to seek out resources and guidance, the advent of the internet has made it easier than ever. You can now find information, advice, and inspiration from successful individuals in your field of interest with just a few clicks. Whether through online articles, videos, or virtual interactions, there are numerous ways to continue feeding your greatness and making progress toward your dreams.

Remember, the key is to maintain the habit of daily effort. By continually feeding your talents and aspirations, you set yourself on a path to success and peace of mind. Your uniqueness is as valuable as the towering bamboo tree, and your greatness deserves the same level of dedicated effort.

Daily nurturing of your gifts and talents puts you in one of two positions: either you are cultivating growth and moving closer to your goals or you are actively living out your dreams as a result of your persistent efforts. The beauty of having a vision for your future is that, with consistent daily care, you can be confident that your dreams will eventually become a reality. By committing to the daily process of watering your greatness, you can find profound peace, knowing that every step you take brings you closer to achieving your full potential.

Lesson #18
Reflections

_____

_____

_____

_____

_____

_____

_____

_____

_____

_____

_____

_____

_____

_____

_____

_____

_____

_____

Part VII

WHEN IT'S ALL
SAID AND DONE

JUST KEEP LIVING

Virginia Woolf said, "you cannot find peace by avoiding life." There are some profound lessons about life that only unfold through the simple act of living. These moments will defy your careful planning, and life will sometimes present you with questions for which there are no immediate answers. But that's perfectly fine. Certain experiences have a way of shattering our established perspectives, no matter how meticulously we've prepared for the path ahead.

If you just keep living, extraordinary events—both awe-inspiring and, at times, seemingly unbearable—will grace your journey. Life will invariably present situations you would never voluntarily choose, yet they will shape you in ways that compel growth and adaptation. Through my years of working with countless individuals, I've observed that when life's storms inevitably strike, there is often a reservoir of resilience and endurance within us, one we may not have known existed. It is precisely in these moments that we are reminded of the importance of embracing life one day at a time, while leaning into the principles that this book has sought to illuminate.

If you keep living, life will teach you principles that offer peace amid the uncertainties and upheavals we encounter. This peace surpasses understanding; it provides an anchor amidst life's turbulence, granting you mental fortitude while fostering stability in other aspects of your existence. These principles hold the power to ground you, offering a tranquility that is not contingent upon the fleeting distractions of the world—a peace that no external force can diminish.

In the face of life's challenges and transitions, these key principles will allow you to confront them with serenity, while also equipping you with the strength and confidence to seize the opportunities of today. This inner calm, this unwavering sense of purpose, will not only sustain you but propel you forward with grace and resilience.

Lesson #19
Reflections

_____

_____

_____

_____

_____

_____

_____

_____

_____

_____

_____

_____

_____

_____

_____

_____

_____

DON'T LET THEM DIE TWICE

No matter who you are, there will come a time when you experience the profound loss of someone who held a unique and irreplaceable place in your life. The bonds we form with certain individuals are so deep, they almost seem to carry a piece of our very essence within them. And if you keep living long enough, you will inevitably face the heartbreak of losing one of these cherished souls to death. When that time comes, I urge you to take life one day at a time. This is not the moment to agonize over how you'll carry on without them, but rather to focus on the strength you need for today. The comfort lies in the fact that with time, the weight of the loss lightens. For now, your task is to live in the present—letting time do its healing work. But whatever you do, don't let them die twice.

During the time you shared with this remarkable person, you forged a connection that defies explanation—an intimacy that others may never fully grasp. You allow them to die twice when you stop living the life they so deeply valued. Remember, they would never want to witness your spirit diminish because of their absence. You let them die twice when their departure becomes a justification for retreating from the people who still cherish you and from the life that still holds meaning. You know the memories you shared, the lessons learned, and the wisdom they imparted. And perhaps you are one of the few who can carry forward the legacy of who they were and what they stood for. Honor their memory by living out the values they instilled in you, letting their life continue through yours.

Lastly, don't let them die twice because of disbelief. Many parents or those who have been around infants will recall moments when a baby appears to be engaging with someone unseen, someone beyond the visible realm. Let this remind you that just because you can no longer see your loved one, their presence can still be felt.

Do not allow their second death to be caused by your surrendering everything that once brought you joy and meaning in their company. If you went hunting together, keep hunting! If you played golf, keep swinging—perhaps you'll even reach that score you both were chasing. If you danced, keep moving to the rhythm you once shared. If you bowled, keep knocking down those pins. If you baked together, keep creating in the kitchen. Whatever the activity, continue it, one day at a time. In these moments, the joy of your bond can still flourish. Even in the face of great loss, you can experience a peace that surpasses understanding when you choose not to let them die twice.

Bonus Lesson #20
Reflections

_____

_____

_____

_____

_____

_____

_____

_____

_____

_____

_____

_____

_____

_____

_____

_____

_____

_____

ABOUT THE AUTHOR

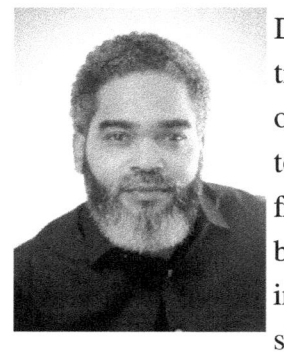 D. L. Jones is a worldwide leader, trainer, author, and professional with over 25 years of experience working to help women, men and children from all backgrounds become the best version of themselves. He has inspired millions through his professional and leadership experiences in Government and Family Services, Community Organizations, The Juvenile Justice System, Religious Organizations, Prisons, and Educational Institutions. D.L. Jones is a recipient of the United States Navy and Marine Corps "Achievement Medal" and he has successfully implemented and facilitated family and male engagement programs in numerous cities throughout the United States. D.L. Jones is a national fatherhood speaker and trainer and CEO of Strategic Engagement Systems LLC, specializing in providing two-generational whole-family learning experiences.

www.ingramcontent.com/pod-product-compliance
Lightning Source LLC
Chambersburg PA
CBHW051539120626
46551CB00013B/1300